contents

The authors would like to acknowledge the following: Contributors, reviewing and rewriting: Jacque Ryan (previous edition); Tracy Flenady (4th edition)
Voluntary reviewers: Judith Applegarth, Patrick Applegarth, Lea Vieth, Lori Nancarrow, Bree Walker (3rd edition); Jennifer Chappell and Lydia Mainey (4th edition)

24-hour clock

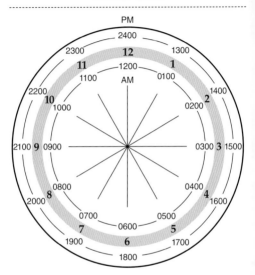

When reporting, charting or ordering any aspect of patient care in health care settings, a 24-hour clock should be used. This reduces the confusion surrounding morning and afternoon times and is particularly important for medication administration orders.

Protecting yourself and the patient

In line with contemporary nursing practice, clinicians must do all they can to reduce harm and improve patient outcomes.[1]

Nurses have a responsibility to implement effective infection control strategies, namely standard and transmission-based precautions.[2–4]

■ STANDARD PRECAUTIONS

These include:
- hand hygiene
- use of personal protective equipment
- safe use and disposal of sharps
- aseptic non-touch technique
- reprocessing of reusable medical equipment and instruments
- respiratory hygiene and cough etiquette
- routine environmental cleaning
- waste management
- appropriate handling of linen.

■ TRANSMISSION-BASED PRECAUTIONS

Used in addition to standard precautions, these include:[2]
- contact precautions

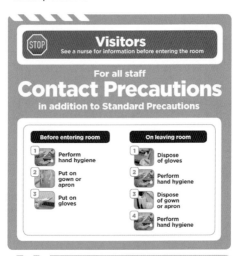

(STOP)
Visitors
See a nurse for information before entering the room

For all staff
Contact Precautions
in addition to Standard Precautions

Before entering room

1. Perform hand hygiene
2. Put on gown or apron
3. Put on gloves

On leaving room

1. Dispose of gloves
2. Perform hand hygiene
3. Dispose of gown or apron
4. Perform hand hygiene

Standard Precautions

And **always** follow these **standard precautions**

- Perform hand hygiene before and after every patient contact
- Use PPE when risk of body fluid exposure

- Use and dispose of sharps safely
- Perform routine environmental cleaning
- Clean and reprocess shared patient equipment

- Follow respiratory hygiene and cough etiquette
- Use aseptic technique
- Handle and dispose of waste and used linen safely

- droplet precautions

Visitors
See a nurse for information before entering the room

For all staff

Droplet Precautions

in addition to Standard Precautions

Before entering room	On leaving room
1 Perform hand hygiene	**1** Dispose of mask
2 Put on a surgical mask	**2** Perform hand hygiene

Standard Precautions

And **always** follow these **standard precautions**

- Perform hand hygiene before and after every patient contact
- Use PPE when risk of body fluid exposure

- Use and dispose of sharps safely
- Perform routine environmental cleaning
- Clean and reprocess shared patient equipment

- Follow respiratory hygiene and cough etiquette
- Use aseptic technique
- Handle and dispose of waste and used linen safely

AUSTRALIAN COMMISSION
ON SAFETY AND QUALITY IN HEALTH CARE

- airborne precautions.

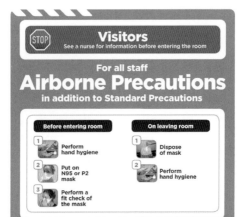

■ OTHER PRECAUTIONS

Cytotoxic—strict adherence to organisational policy.[5]

■ HAND HYGIENE

5 moments of hand hygiene[6]

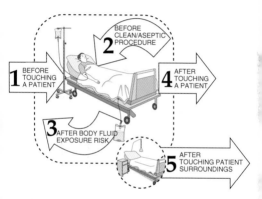

■ PERSONAL PROTECTIVE EQUIPMENT (PPE)

PPE includes gloves, masks, protective eyewear, aprons/gowns and face shields.

Examples of application of PPE:

- Wear *gloves* when there is a potential for soiling your hands with body fluids. Always wash your hands when you remove your gloves.
- Wear a *mask* when there is a risk of inhaling or coming into contact with body fluids.
- Wear *protective eyewear/face shields* when there is a potential for being splashed, splattered or sprayed with body fluids.
- Wear a *plastic apron* when there is a risk of body fluids coming into contact with your clothes.
- Always adhere to organisation protocol for specific conditions.

Sequence for donning PPE[7]

Steps to put on personal protective equipment (PPE)

1
Always put on essential required PPE when handling either a suspected, probable or confirmed case of viral haemorrhagic fever.

2
The dressing and undressing of PPE should be supervised by another trained member of the team.

3 Gather all the necessary items of PPE beforehand. Put on the scrub suit in the changing room.

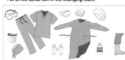

4 Put on rubber boots. If not available, make sure you have closed, puncture and fluid resistant shoes and put on overshoes.

OR, IF BOOTS UNAVAILABLE

5 Place the impermeable gown over the scrubs.

6 Put on face protection:
6a Put on a medical mask.

6b Put on goggles or a face shield.

7
If available, put a head cover on at this time.

8 Perform hand hygiene.

9 Put on gloves* (over cuff).

10 If an impermeable gown is not available, place waterproof apron over gown.

While wearing PPE:
- Avoid touching or adjusting PPE
- Change gloves between patients
- Remove gloves if they become torn or damaged
- Perform hand hygiene before putting on new gloves

* Use **double** gloves if any strenuous activity (e.g. carrying a patient or handling a dead body) or tasks in which contact with blood and body fluids are anticipated. Use **heavy duty/rubber gloves** for environmental cleaning and waste management.

World Health Organization

Sequence for doffing PPE[7]

Steps to **remove** personal protective equipment (PPE)

1 Remove waterproof apron and dispose of safely. If the apron is to be reused, place it in a container with disinfectant.

2 If wearing overshoes, remove them with your gloves still on (If wearing rubber boots, see step 4).

3 Remove gown and gloves and roll inside-out and dispose of safely.

4 If wearing rubber boots, remove them (ideally using the boot remover) without touching them with your hands. Place them in a container with disinfectant.

5 Perform hand hygiene.

6 If wearing a head cover, remove it now (from behind the head).

7 Remove face protection:
7a Remove face shield or goggles (from behind the head). Place eye protection in a separate container for reprocessing.

7b Remove mask from behind the head. When removing mask, untie the bottom string first and the top string next.

8 Perform hand hygiene.

World Health Organization

■ BODY FLUIDS EXPOSURE[8]

Immediately

- Wash skin sites with soap and water.
- Irrigate mucous membranes and eyes (remove contact lenses) with water or saline.
- If it is a sharps injury, wash with soap and water.

Next

- Report the exposure to your supervisor.
- Adhere to the organisation's protocol. This may involve presenting to either the emergency department of a hospital or a general practitioner.

■ MOVING PATIENTS SAFELY[9]

Think ...

S	Stick to organisation policy and procedure.
A	Assess environment, patient and mobility plan, including patient dependency code, before any transfer.
F	Follow safe practice—plan the transfer, use required resources, communicate with the patient, implement correct techniques.
E	Evaluate and document.

Example of bed mobility codes

I	**Independent:** Patient doesn't need assistance with technique/transfer, but may use equipment to assist themself.
S	**Supervision:** Patient needs to be supervised and/or prompted verbally with technique/transfer; may be with or without self-help aids.

(Continued)

| A | **Assistance:** Patient needs assistance of one or more people and/or equipment to complete the transfer/technique. The patient can understand and cooperate, and is physically able to perform part of the activity. |
| TD | **Totally dependent:** The patient is not able to understand or cooperate, or is unable to physically assist with the transfer/technique and needs equipment. Two or more persons are required and patient-handling equipment is essential. |

Examples of mobility equipment codes

H	Hoist	MWC	Manual wheelchair
SS	Slide sheet	PWC	Powered wheelchair
2WW	Two-wheeled walker	R	Rollator
PS	Patient slide	WB	Walk belt
QS	Quad stick	WS	Walking stick

■ FALLS PREVENTION[1, 10]

Falls are a major concern and occur in health care facilities daily. The Australian Commission on Safety and Quality in Health Care (ACSQHC) has developed various tools for clinicians to utilise in order to reduce the risk of falls occurring.[10–11] Nurses have a responsibility for falls prevention and harm minimisation. Responsibilities include:

- Undertake a risk assessment.
- Document the falls risk status.
- Implement strategies to minimise falls.

Example of a falls risk assessment and management tool[12]

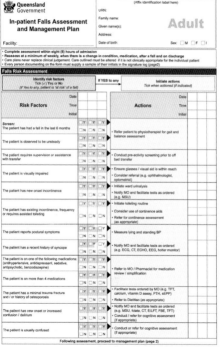

Queensland Government

In-patient Falls Assessment and Management Plan

(Affix identification label here)

URN:
Family name:
Given name(s):
Address:
Date of birth:

Adult

Sex: ☐ M ☐ F ☐ I

Facility:

- Complete assessment within eight (8) hours of admission
- Reassess at a minimum of weekly, when there is a change in condition, medication, after a fall and on discharge
- Care plans never replace clinical judgement. Care outlined must be altered if it is not clinically appropriate for the individual patient
- Every person documenting on the form must supply a sample of their initials in the signature log (page2)

Falls Risk Assessment

Identify risk factors — Tick (✓) Yes or No (If Yes to any, patient is 'at risk' of a fall)	If YES to any	Initiate actions — Tick when actioned (if indicated)			
Risk Factors		**Actions**	Date		
			Time		
			Initial		
Screen: The patient has had a fall in the last 6 months	☐Y ☐Y ☐Y ☐N ☐N ☐N	• Refer patient to physiotherapist for gait and balance assessment			
The patient is observed to be unsteady	☐Y ☐Y ☐Y ☐N ☐N ☐N				
The patient requires supervision or assistance with transfer	☐Y ☐Y ☐Y ☐N ☐N ☐N	• Conduct pre-activity screening prior to off bed transfer			
The patient is visually impaired	☐Y ☐Y ☐Y ☐N ☐N ☐N	• Ensure glasses / visual aid is within reach • Consider referral (e.g. ophthalmologist, optometrist)			
The patient has new onset incontinence	☐Y ☐Y ☐Y ☐N ☐N ☐N	• Initiate ward urinalysis • Notify MO and facilitate tests as ordered (e.g. MSU)			
The patient has existing incontinence, frequency or requires assisted toileting	☐Y ☐Y ☐Y ☐N ☐N ☐N	• Initiate toileting routine • Consider use of continence aids • Refer for continence assessment (as appropriate)			
The patient reports postural symptoms	☐Y ☐Y ☐Y ☐N ☐N ☐N	• Measure lying and standing BP			
The patient has a recent history of syncope	☐Y ☐Y ☐Y ☐N ☐N ☐N	• Notify MO and facilitate tests as ordered (e.g. ECG, CT, ECHO, holter monitor)			
The patient is on one of the following medications: (antihypertensive, antidepressant, sedative, antipsychotic, benzodiazepine)	☐Y ☐Y ☐Y ☐N ☐N ☐N	• Refer to MO / Pharmacist for medication review / simplification			
The patient is on more than 4 medications	☐Y ☐Y ☐Y ☐N ☐N ☐N				
The patient has a minimal trauma fracture and / or history of osteoporosis	☐Y ☐Y ☐Y ☐N ☐N ☐N	• Facilitate tests ordered by MO (e.g. TFT, calcium, vitamin D assay, PTH, sEPP) • Refer to Dietitian (as appropriate)			
The patient has new onset or increased confusion / delirium	☐Y ☐Y ☐Y ☐N ☐N ☐N	• Notify MO and facilitate tests as ordered (e.g. MSU, folate, CT, E/LFT, FBE, TFT) • Conduct / refer for cognitive assessment (if appropriate)			
The patient is usually confused	☐Y ☐Y ☐Y ☐N ☐N ☐N	• Conduct or refer for cognitive assessment (if appropriate)			

Following assessment, proceed to management plan (page 2)

Queensland Government

In-patient Falls Assessment and Management Plan

Adult

(Affix identification label here)

URN:

Family name:

Given name(s):

Address:

Date of birth: Sex: ☐ M ☐ F ☐ I

- Complete within eight (8) hours of admission
- Review management plan at a minimum daily and document as per local policy
- Initial when strategies are implemented
- V indicates a variance from clinical care and must be documented in the clinical notes

Falls Prevention Management Plan

All care givers who initial are to sign signature log   ☞ Key ◆ Allied Health ■ Medical ▲ Nursing ☺ Pharmacy

Category	☞		Date			
			Time			
Communication	▲	In partnership with patient and / or carer discuss falls risk factors and develop falls prevention plan				
		Provide written falls prevention information (e.g. *Stay On Your Feet® BE SAFE* brochure)				
		Communicate patients 'at risk' status at bedside handover				
		Instruct patient to call for assistance when getting out of bed / mobilising (if required)				
Environment / Equipment	▲	Orientate patient to surroundings, routine and location of bathroom and toilet				
		Ensure clutter free and safe environment (e.g. night time lighting)				
		Ensure the bed height and position are suitable for the patient's needs				
		Apply bed brakes correctly				
		Ensure bed rails are at appropriate height for patient's needs				
		Keep buzzer in reach; educate patient on buzzer usage				
		Keep patient's routine belongings within reach				
		Keep patient's mobility aid in reach if applicable				
		Review patient footwear and / or foot problems				
Observations	▲	Ensure frequent rounding and surveillance				
		Consider supervision during toileting / showering / mobilisation				
		Ensure suitable toileting protocols are in place				
Other Care (specify)	▲ ◆ ■ ☺					
Discharge Planning / Education	▲	Provide information on falls risk factors and prevention strategies				
		Refer to OT for ADL and home assessment				
		Complete nursing discharge summary and facilitate referrals				

Signature Log

Initial	Print name	Designation	Signature	Initial	Print name	Designation	Signature

The 5 Bs of falls prevention
1. Belongings within reach (e.g. spectacles)
2. Buzzer within reach
3. Brakes on
4. Bed low
5. Bedrails only if prescribed; otherwise, bedrails down

■ VENOUS THROMBOEMBOLISM (VTE) PREVENTION[13]

Venous thromboembolism (VTE) includes both deep vein thrombosis (DVT) and pulmonary embolism (PE). Many hospitalised patients may have risk factors for VTE.

Risk factors include:
- age > 60
- pregnancy and the peurperium
- previous VTE/family history
- varicose veins
- marked obesity
- leg injury requiring surgery or prolonged immobilisation
- prolonged surgery
- prolonged immobility
- general anaesthesia
- myocardial infarction
- stroke with immobility.

Strategies for prevention
- Conduct a risk assessment and document.
- Consider a patient review by medical staff for anticoagulant prophylaxis.
- Consider mechanical prophylaxis, including graduated compression stockings (GCS) and intermittent pneumatic compression devices (ICP).

- Promote mobilisation.
- Immediately report and seek help when the patient complains of pain/swelling in lower legs combined with dyspnoea or chest pain.

■ SUDDEN INFANT DEATH SYNDROME (SIDS): SAFE SLEEPING[14]

When caring for infants in a hospital setting, nurses should be aware of the following SIDS risk reduction factors:

S	**S**leep baby on back from birth
I	**I**n their own safe environment (e.g. for first 6–12 months should be in own cot beside parent's bed with safe mattress and bedding)
D	**D**on't cover face or overheat baby
S	**S**moke-free zone (before and after birth)

Medication safety[1, 15]

In order to reduce the incidence of medication error, the ACSQHC has developed medication safety guidelines.[14] The following tips should be considered when adhering to the ACSQHC guidelines, as well as specific organisational requirements.

■ FIVE RIGHTS AND MORE

FIVE RIGHTS AND MORE	THREE CHECKS
1. Right medication 2. Right dose 3. Right time 4. Right route 5. Right patient And more: • Right effect • Right to refuse • Right form • Right patient education • Right documentation • Right assessment • Right evaluation	1. Check the label when getting the drug from storage. 2. Check the drug label with the drug order. 3. Recheck the drug order and drug after dispensing *but* prior to administration.

■ MEDICATION ORDERS[16]

MEDICATION ORDER INCLUSIONS	MEDICATION CHART INCLUSIONS
• date ordered	• patient's name
• route	• unique record (UR) number
• generic drug name	• date of birth
• dose ordered	• address
• date and time drug to be administered	• weight
• prescriber's signature and printed name	• allergies

Do not administer a medication when:

- any element of the order is missing
- the order is not legible
- the order is not safe—for example: dose, route and timing is incorrect; the patient is allergic to the medication; the medication interacts with another, including intravenous fluids; or the patient's condition may be impacted in a negative way as a result of the action of the medication that is ordered (e.g. the patient is in a hypotensive state and is ordered regular antihypertensives).

■ MEDICATION SAFETY TIPS

- Check allergies (ask patient, check for allergy band, check medication chart).
- If unfamiliar with a medication's action, look it up.
- Check decimal points.
- Always question large doses.
- Be aware of the risk of error with medications that look alike and sound alike.
- Consider the risk of errors if you are administering medications when hungry, angry, late or tired (HALT).
- Use caution with high-risk medications—insulin, heparin, narcotics, cytotoxics, antibiotics, potassium.
- Never leave unadministered medications unattended.
- Do not administer anything that you have not prepared yourself.

- Always check paediatric medications against mg/kg and recommended dose according to paediatric medication dosing guidelines (online or hard copy resources).

Oral medications—safety tips

- Make sure the patient is sitting up.
- Use oral dispensing devices for oral suspensions to reduce the risk of administering via the wrong route.
- If working with children, seek their cooperation as well as that of their parents/caregivers.
- Paediatric medication orders require two persons present from the point of preparation to administration.
- Make sure the patient is capable of swallowing.
- Check the patient has fluid to swallow the medication.
- Measure oral liquid medicine at eye level, with the measure cup on a flat surface.
- Do not administer oral medication if the patient:
  — is sedated
  — has no gag/swallowing reflex
  — is vomiting.

Injections—safety tips

- All injections require a second-person check (a student nurse cannot be the second checker).
- Be aware of onset of action and side effects.
- Know the landmarks for intramuscular (IM) and subcutaneous.

- Use the correct needle and syringe.
- Never recap a needle.
- Dispose of the needle and syringe appropriately.
- Be aware that the volumes of injections alter in children depending on their age and muscle mass.

Intramuscular injection landmarks

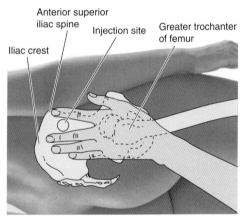

Ventrogluteal site

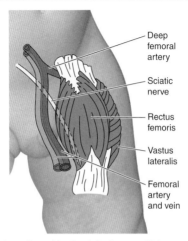

Vastus lateralis muscle of an infant's upper thigh

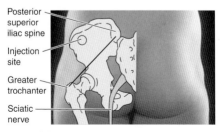

Dorsogluteal site

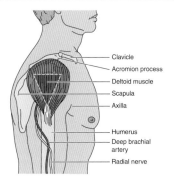

Deltoid muscle of the upper arm

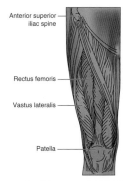

Rectus femoris muscle of the upper right thigh

■ MEDICATION ADMINISTRATION AND STUDENT NURSES

Students should only administer medications if:

- organisation policy permits
- tertiary requirements permit
- the skill is within the student's scope
- the student is:
  - — prepared
  - — only administering to patients within their care
  - — directly supervised by a Registered Nurse.

■ ABBREVIATIONS USED IN MEDICATION ADMINISTRATION[16]

Dose frequency or timing

INTENDED MEANING	ACCEPTABLE TERMS OR ABBREVIATIONS
in the morning	morning, mane
midday	midday
night	night, nocte
twice a day	bd
three times a day	tds
four times a day	qid
every 4 hours	every 4 hours, 4 hourly, 4 hrly
every 6 hours	every 6 hours, 6 hourly, 6 hrly
every 8 hours	every 8 hours, 8 hourly, 8 hrly
once a week	once a week and specific, the exact day in full

(Continued)

three times a week	three times a week and specific, exact days in full
when required	prn
immediately	stat
before food	before food
after food	after food
with food	with food

Reason for nurse not administering

Absent	A
Fasting	F
Refused—notify Dr	R
Vomiting	V
On leave	L
Not available—obtain supply or contact Dr	N
Withheld—enter reason in clinical record	W
Self-administering	S
The code MUST be circled.	

Route of administration

INTENDED MEANING	ACCEPTABLE TERMS OR ABBREVIATIONS
inhale, inhalation	inhale, inhalation
intramuscular	IM

intranasal	intranasal
intravenous	IV
irrigation	irrigation
left	left
nebulised	NEB
nasogastric	NG
per oral	PO
percutaneous enteral gastrostomy	PEG
per rectum	PR
per vagina	PV
peripherally inserted central catheter	PICC
right	right
subcutaneous	subcut
sublingual	subling
topical	topical

Units of measure and concentration

INTENDED MEANING	ACCEPTABLE TERMS OR ABBREVIATIONS
grams	g
International unit(s)	International unit(s)
unit(s)	unit(s)

(Continued)

litre(s)	L
milligram(s)	mg
millilitre(s)	mL
microgram(s)	microgram, microg
percentage	%
millimole	mmol

Dose forms

INTENDED MEANING	ACCEPTABLE TERMS OR ABBREVIATIONS
capsule	cap
cream	cream
ear drops	ear drops
ear ointment	ear ointment
eye drops	eye drops
injection	inj
metered dose inhaler	metered dose inhaler, inhaler, MDI
ointment	ointment, oint
pessary	pess
powder	powder
suppository	supp
tablet	tablet, tab
patient-controlled analgesia	PCA

■ PERIPHERAL INTRAVENOUS CATHETER (PIVC) MAINTENANCE[17]

PIVC sites should be reviewed every 8 hours, ensuring that all access sites are assessed for:

- catheter position
- occlusion/patency
- dressing intact.

Assess PIVC sites for the following conditions

CONDITION	INDICATIONS
Phlebitis	<ul><li>erythema</li><li>tenderness</li><li>swelling</li><li>pain</li><li>purulent discharge</li></ul>
Systemic infection	<ul><li>rigor</li><li>fever</li><li>tachycardia</li><li>hypotension</li><li>malaise</li><li>nausea/vomiting</li></ul>
Infiltration/extravasation	<ul><li>Insertion site:<ul><li>cool skin</li><li>blanched, taut skin</li><li>oedema</li><li>IV fluid leaking</li><li>burning/stinging pain</li><li>redness</li></ul></li></ul>

■ METRIC SYSTEM AND SYMBOLS

Metric system

VOLUME

1 litre (L)	=	1000 millilitres (mL)

MASS

1 kilogram (kg)	=	1000 grams (g)
1 gram (g)	=	1000 milligrams (mg)
1 milligram (mg)	=	1000 micrograms (µg)

LENGTH

1 kilometre (km)	=	1000 metres (m)
1 metre (m)	=	100 centimetres (cm)
1 centimetre (cm)	=	10 millimetres (mm)

EXAMPLE OF EQUIVALENCES

0.2 kilograms	=	200 grams
0.2 grams	=	200 milligrams
0.2 milligrams	=	200 micrograms
0.2 litres	=	200 millilitres

Decimals, percentages and fractions

DECIMALS	PERCENTAGES	FRACTIONS
0.01	1%	1/100
0.05	5%	5/100
0.20	20%	20/100
0.30	30%	30/100
0.40	40%	40/100
0.50	50%	50/100
0.60	60%	60/100

0.70	70%	70/100
0.80	80%	80/100
0.90	90%	90/100
1.00	100%	100/100

■ DRUG CALCULATIONS/FORMULAS

Drug dosages

$$\text{Amount required} = \frac{\text{strength required}}{\text{strength in stock}} \times \frac{\text{volume}}{1}$$

OR

$$\text{Amount required} = \frac{\text{required strength}}{\text{stored strength}} \times \frac{\text{volume}}{1}$$

Intravenous infusions

$$\text{Rate (drops per minute)} = \frac{\text{volume to be infused}}{\text{time in hours}} \times \frac{\text{drop rate}}{60 \text{ minutes}}$$

(The drop rate is found on the drip set in Australia: macrodrop 20 drops/mL, microdrop 60 drops/mL.)

$$\text{Rate (mL/h)} = \frac{\text{volume (mL)}}{\text{time (hours)}}$$

µg/kg/min: this calculation is a three-step process

$$\frac{\text{ordered dose in µg}}{\text{volume (mL)}} \times \frac{\text{infusion rate (mL/h)}}{60} \times \frac{1}{\text{body weight (kg)}}$$

Drip rates

Drip rates for giving sets where: 20 drops = 1 mL

1000 mL	mL/HR	DROPS/MIN
Over 2 hours	500	167
Over 4 hours	250	83
Over 6 hours	167	55
Over 8 hours	125	42
Over 10 hours	100	33
Over 12 hours	83	28

■ DRUG NAME ENDINGS AND RELATED INFORMATION[17]

SUFFIX	DRUG GROUP	EXAMPLE
Anaesthetics (local)		
-caine	Esters	Procaine
		Amethocaine
	Amides	Lignocaine
		Prilocaine
Antibiotics		
-illin	Penicillin	Ampicillin
-cycline	Tetracyclines	Doxycycline
-cin	Aminoglycosides	Gentamycin
-mycin	Macrolides	Erythromycin
-oxacin	Quinolones	Ciprofloxacin

Cardiac/Antihypertensive drugs

-olol	Beta blockers	Propranolol
-dipine	Calcium channel blockers	Felodipine
		Nifedipine
		Amlodipine
-pril	Angiotensin converting enzyme (ACE) inhibitors	Captopril
		Enalapril
-sartan	AT_1-receptor blockers	Losartan
		Irbesartan

Diuretics

-ide	Loop diuretic	Frusemide

Fibrinolytics

-inase	Enzyme	Streptokinase
		Urokinase

Neuromuscular blockers

-ium	Depolarising or non-competitive blockers	Suxamethonium
	Competitive blockers	Atracurium
		Pancuronium

Oral hypoglycaemics

-ide	Sulfonylureas	Gliclazide
		Gilbencalmide

Sedatives/Anxiolytics

-azepam	Benzodiazepines	Nitrazepam

■ HIGH-RISK MEDICINES RESOURCE (APINCHS)[18]

ALL HIGH-RISK MEDICINES REQUIRE AN INDEPENDENT SECOND CHECK		
A	Anti-infectives	• Administered timely and monitored appropriately
P	Potassium and other electrolytes	• Potassium is NOT added to any premixed bag • Check IV patency prior to administering • Usually infused at maximum rate of 20 mmol/hr
I	Insulin	• Cannot be administered without a valid order • Insulin is measured in international units
N	Narcotics and other sedatives	• Includes all schedule 8 (S8) and restricted schedule (RS4) medications • Check patient's sedation score prior to administering
C	Chemotherapeutic agents	• Use cytotoxic precautions when administering • Patients are 'hot' for 7 days post cytotoxic administration • Pregnant staff not to handle cytotoxic medications or waste

H	Heparin and other anticoagulants	• Includes heparin, enoxaparin, danaparoid, warfarin, rivaroxaban, dabigatran and apixaban • Monitor for signs of bleeding • For warfarin, check patient's international normalised ratio (INR)

S	Systems	• Familiarise yourself with best practice recommendations for medication delivery systems:
		  ○ oral syringes
		  ○ infusion pumps
		  ○ injectables
		  ○ injection landmarks
		  ○ drug calculations

■ DRUGS AND ANTIDOTES[19]

DRUG OVERDOSE	ANTIDOTE
Benzodiazepine	Flumazenil
Paracetamol	Acetylcysteine
Warfarin	Vitamin K_1 (phytomenaidone)
Atropine	Physostigmine salicylate
Heparin	Protamine sulfate

(Continued)

Anticholinesterase	Atropine, pralidoxime iodide
Iron poisoning	Desferrioxamine; Deferiprone; Desferasirox
Narcotic	Naloxone
Digoxin	Antidogin antibodies; Atropine; Phenytoin; Disodium edetale
Non-specific poisons (except cyanide, iron, lithium, caustics and alcohol)	Activated charcoal

Oxygen concentration delivery[20]

DELIVERY APPARATUS	OXYGEN FLOW RATE (L/MIN)	APPROXIMATE % OF OXYGEN
Room air/no apparatus		21
Nasal prongs	1–2 3–4 5–6	24–28 32–36 40–44
Hudson mask	6–8	44–60
Non-rebreathing mask	10–15	85–95 (bag must be inflated)

Note: Be aware of variations in flow rates for children—check with organisation policy.

Fluid balance

■ USEFUL MEASUREMENTS FOR FLUID BALANCE CHARTS

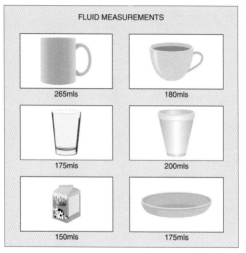

FLUID MEASUREMENTS

265mls	180mls
175mls	200mls
150mls	175mls

Fluid container volumes

■ FLUID BALANCE SAFETY TIPS

- If output is > input, the patient is in a negative balance.
- If input is > output, the patient is in a positive balance.
- Make sure patients and family/caregivers know they are on a fluid balance chart.
- Always ask the patient input and output when updating the fluid balance chart.
- The urinary output should be >0.5 mL/kg/h.
- Report urinary output of <30 mL/h.
- Gain or loss of 1 kg equates to 1 L of fluid retained or lost.

■ CLASSIFICATION OF URINE OUTPUT[21]

- Anuria: no urine output.
- Oliguria: less than 400 mL/day.
- Polyuria: greater than 2500 mL/day.

■ FLUID LOSSES

The table below indicates appropriate fluid choices for ongoing fluid losses.

Properties of some common fluids[22]

TYPE OF FLUID	SODIUM mmol/L	POTASSIUM mmol/L	CHLORIDE mmol/L	GLUCOSE g/L
Sodium chloride 0.9%	154	0	154	0
Compound sodium lactate (Hartmann's)	129	5	109	0

Plasma-lyte 148 in water	140	5	98	0
0.3% sodium chloride and 3.3% glucose	51	0	51	33
5% glucose	0	0	0	50

■ **FLUID REDISTRIBUTION PROPERTIES**[22]

ISOTONIC SOLUTIONS	HYPOTONIC SOLUTIONS	HYPERTONIC SOLUTIONS
The same osmotic pressure as body plasma	Less osmotic pressure than plasma	More osmotic pressure than plasma
<ul><li>whole blood</li><li>Hartmann's</li><li>4% glucose with 0.18% sodium chloride</li><li>5% glucose</li><li>0.9% sodium chloride.</li></ul>	<ul><li>water</li><li>0.45% sodium chloride</li><li>0.3% sodium chloride</li><li>4% glucose.</li></ul>	<ul><li>25% mannitol</li><li>10% glucose</li><li>5–10% glucose combined with 0.2–0.9% sodium chloride</li><li>20% albumin.</li></ul>

■ BODY WEIGHT METHOD FOR CALCULATING DAILY MAINTENANCE FLUIDS

Paediatrics[23]

WEIGHT	FLUID mL/DAY	mL/HOUR
3–10 kg	100 × wt	4 × wt
10–20 kg	1000 plus 50 × (wt–10)	40 plus 2 × (wt–10)
>20 kg	1500 plus 20 × (wt–20)	60 plus 1 × (wt–20)
Note: 100 mL/hour (2400 mL/day) is the normal maximum amount.		

Patient assessments

Recognising and responding to patients who are clinically deteriorating is an integral aspect of nursing care. For prompt and appropriate action to occur, clinicians must use all available resources to identify physiological, cognitive and mental changes that herald clinical decline.[24]

■ VITAL SIGNS

- Temperature (T): normal 36.5–37.1 PO
  Note: Infant's temperature should be maintained >36.5.
- Heart rate (HR): rate, rhythm, strength regularity
- Respiratory rate (RR): rate, depth, pattern, use of accessory muscles
- Blood pressure (BP)

- Mean arterial pressure (MAP): {(systolic BP − diastolic BP)/3} + diastolic BP
- Blood oxygen saturation as measured by pulse oximeter (SpO_2)

■ VITAL SIGNS: NORMAL RANGES[25]

AGE (years)	RESPIRATORY RATE (breaths/ min)	HEART RATE (beats/ min)	SYSTOLIC BLOOD PRESSURE (mm Hg)	OXYGEN SATURATION
1 mth–1	50–53	100–190	72–104	>95%
1–2	22–37	98–140	86–106	>95%
3–5	20–28	80–120	89–112	>95%
6–11	18–25	75–118	97–120	>95%
12–15	12-20	60–100	110–131	>95%
Adult	12–20	60–100	100–130	>95%

■ EARLY WARNING SYSTEMS (ADULT)

Early warning systems are used to track patients' vital signs by allocating points to each parameter measured. If the total value from the combined vital signs reaches a pre-determined score, clinicians are required to carry out certain actions designed to prevent adverse outcomes.

Adult		Date									
		Time									
Respiratory Rate (breaths / min) Measure for a full minute	E	≥35									E
	3	30–34									3
	1	25–29									1
		21–24									
	0	17–20									0
		13–16									
	1	9–12									1
	E	<8									E
O₂ Saturation (%)		≥98									0
		95–97									
	1	90–94									1
	2	85–89									2
	3	≤84									3
Oxygen* (L / min or % delivered) *If on HF / NIV use % delivered	E	NFM									E
	3	>11	>50%								3
	2	>5–11	>40–50%							2
	1	2–5	28–40%							1
	0	<2	<28%							0
Mode	FM Face mask	NP Nasal prongs	NFM² High flow nasal prongs								Circle
	HF High flow	NIV Non-invasive									
	NIV Non-invasive	RA Room air									
Actual FIO₂ on Device Screen											
High Flow L/min on Device Screen											Actual BP
Blood Pressure (mmHg) ∨ ∧ Score systolic BP		≥200									≥200
		190s									190s
		180s									180s
		170s									170s
		160s									160s
		150s									150s
		140s									140s
		130s									130s
		120s									120s
		110s									110s
		100s									100s
		90s									90s
		80s									80s
		70s									70s
		60s									60s
Systolic BP score											
Heart Rate (beats / min)	E	≥140									E
	3	130s									3
	2	120s									2
	1	110s									1
		100s									
		90s									
	0	80s									0
		70s									
		60s									
		50s									
	2	40s									2
	E	30s									E
Temperature (°C)	2	≥39.5									2
	1	38.5–39.4									1
		38–38.4									
		37.5–37.9									
	0	37–37.4									0
		36.1–36.9									
	1	35.1–36									1
	2	34.1–35									2
	3	≤34									3
Consciousness If necessary, wake patient before scoring	0	Alert									0
	1	Voice									1
	4	New confusion / agitation	4	4	4	4	4	4	4	4	4
		Pain									
	E	Unresponsive									E
Modifications in use	M										
TOTAL Q-ADDS SCORE											
Interventions	(e.g. 'A')										
Initials											

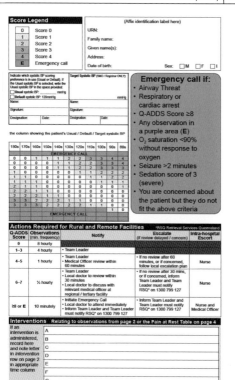

Score Legend

0	Score 0
1	Score 1
2	Score 2
3	Score 3
4	Score 4
E	Emergency call

(Affix identification label here)

URN:

Family name:

Given name(s):

Address:

Date of birth: Sex: ☐ M ☐ F ☐ I

Indicate which systolic BP scoring preference you'd prefer (Usual or Default). If the Usual systolic BP is selected, write the Usual systolic BP in the space provided.

☐ Usual systolic BP: _____ mmHg
☐ Default systolic BP: 120mmHg

Target Systolic BP (SMO / Register ONLY)

_____ mmHg

Name:

Signature:

Designation: Date:

Name:

Signature:

Designation: Date:

Emergency call if:
- Airway Threat
- Respiratory or cardiac arrest
- Q-ADDS Score ≥8
- Any observation in a purple area (E)
- O₂ saturation <90% without response to oxygen
- Seizure >2 minutes
- Sedation score of 3 (severe)
- You are concerned about the patient but they do not fit the above criteria

the column showing the patient's Usual / Default / Target systolic BP

180s	170s	160s	150s	140s	130s	120s	110s	100s	90s	80s
					EMERGENCY CALL					
0	0	1	1	1	2	2	3	3	4	4
0	0	0	1	1	2	2	3	3	4	
0	0	0	0	1	1	2	2	3	3	
1	0	0	0	0	1	1	2	2	3	
1	1	0	0	0	0	1	1	2	2	
2	1	1	0	0	0	0	1	1		
2	2	1	1	0	0	0	0	0		
2	2	2	1	1	0	0	0	0		
3	3	2	2	1	1	0	0			
3	3	3	2	2	2	1	1	0	0	
									1	0
					EMERGENCY CALL					

Actions Required for Rural and Remote Facilities *RSQ Retrieval Services Queensland*

Q-ADDS Score	Observations (min. frequency)	Notify	Escalate (if review delayed / concern)	Intra-hospital Escort
0	8 hourly			
1–3	4 hourly	• Team Leader		
4–5	1 hourly	• Team Leader • Medical Officer review within 60 minutes	• If no review after 60 minutes, or if concerned, follow local escalation plan	Nurse
6–7	½ hourly	• Team Leader • Local doctor to review within 30 minutes • Local doctor to discuss with relevant medical officer at regional / tertiary facility	• If no review after 30 mins, or if concerned, inform Team Leader and Team Leader must notify RSQ* on 1300 799 127	Nurse
≥8 or E	10 minutely	• Initiate Emergency Call • Local doctor to attend immediately • Inform Team Leader and Team Leader must notify RSQ* on 1300 799 127	• Inform Team Leader and Team Leader must notify RSQ* on 1300 799 127	Nurse and Medical Officer

Interventions Relating to observations from page 2 or the Pain at Rest Table on page 4

If an intervention is administered, record here and note letter in intervention row on page 2 in appropriate time column

A	
B	
C	
D	
E	
F	
G	

Queensland Adult Deterioration Detection System (QADDS)

■ QUICK HEAD-TO-TOE ASSESSMENT

General

Always provide privacy, compare right and left sides, and document and report findings.

Neurological

Look for signs of orientation to time and place.
Record Glasgow Coma Scale (GCS) score as necessary.

Glasgow Coma Scale[26]

Eyes open	Spontaneous	4
	To sound	3
	To pressure	2
	No response	1
Best verbal response	Oriented	5
	Confused	4
	Inappropriate words	3
	Incomprehensible sounds	2
	No response	1
Best motor response	Obeys commands	6
	Localises to pain	5
	Normal flexion	4
	Flexion to pain (decorticate)	3
	Extension to pain (decerebrate)	2
	No response	1

AVPU responsiveness scale[13]

A	Alert
V	Verbal: Responsive to verbal stimuli (consider GCS)
P	Pain: Responsive to central painful stimuli (conduct GCS)
U	Unresponsive

Cardiovascular

- Look at the patient's colour.
- Feel the distal pulses (radial, brachial, pedal) and apical pulse (use stethoscope).
- Feel strength, rhythm and rate of the pulse.
- Feel for oedema in the feet and dependent areas.
- Obtain the blood pressure (unless otherwise indicated).
- Assess capillary refill (normal = <2 seconds).

Respiratory[27]

- Look for respiratory pattern, rate, symmetry, use of accessory muscles, nasal flaring, tracheal tug and patient position. (Does the patient look comfortable breathing? Are they experiencing difficulty?)
- Assess oxygen saturation (normal = >98%).
- Listen for equal air entry to both lungs.
- Listen for noises such as crepitations or wheezes.
- Examine the sputum.
- For children, observe for the following signs of respiratory distress:
  — nasal flaring
  — grunting

- prolonged respiratory phase
- tracheal tug
- sternal recession
- use of accessory muscles
- drooling that is accompanied by a tripod sitting position.

Skin

- Look at the colour, scars or lesions.
- Feel the temperature, moisture, turgor and capillary refill (normal = <2 seconds).
- Assess for oedema, noting:
  — location
  — temperature of skin
  — shape
  — degree that skin remains pitted.

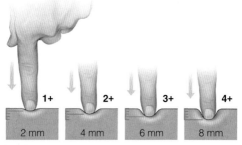

Degree that skin remains pitted[28]

Abdomen

- Look, then listen and then feel.
- Look for distension and scars.
- Listen for bowel sounds (normal sounds occur every 15–20 seconds).
- Percuss:
  — Dullness is a solid organ.
  — Tympany is air-filled.
  — Flatness is muscle or bone.
- Feel for pulsations, masses, tenderness and rigidity.
- Always start in the least painful area.

Extremities

- Look at the colour, movement, warmth, sensation and strength of limbs.
- Feel for swelling or pain in the calf. This may be an indication of thrombosis or thrombophlebitis.
- Look at nail beds for capillary refill or signs of clubbing and discolouration.

Other

Listen to the history of the presenting condition:

- date and time of onset
- causative factors
- action taken to relieve symptoms
- family history
- medications
- social history, employment and family situation
- lifestyle, diet, alcohol and exercise.

■ SIGNS OF STROKE[29]

F	**F**acial weakness: Ask the person to smile.	Is their face symmetrical?
A	**A**rm weakness: Ask the person to raise both arms.	Can they raise both arms?
S	**S**peech difficulty: Ask the person to say a simple sentence.	Can you understand what they are saying?
T	**T**ime to act FAST	Seek medical assistance.

■ SIGNS OF SEPSIS

S	**S**hivering, fever or very cold
E	**E**xtreme pain or general discomfort
P	**P**ale or discoloured skin
S	**S**leepy, difficult to rouse, confused
I	'**I** feel like I might die'
S	**S**hort of breath

■ NEUROVASCULAR ASSESSMENT[13]

ASSESSMENT	UNEXPECTED FINDINGS
Colour	Pallor or cyanosis
Temperature	Cool/Cold/Hot
Capillary refill time	Greater than 4 seconds

Swelling	Significantly swollen
Pain	Presence of moderate to severe pain
Movement	Little or none

■ PAIN ASSESSMENT[13]

When assessing pain, remember PQRST:

	Ask the patient:
P = *Precipitation/Palliation*	What causes the pain? What relieves the pain?
Q = *Quality*	What does the pain feel like? (Is it sharp, stabbing, dull, crushing?)
R = *Region/Radiation*	Where did the pain start? Where does the pain travel to?
S = *Severity*	How bad is the pain? (Use a pain scale: 0 = no pain, 10 = worst pain)
T = *Timing*	When did the pain start? How long does the pain last?

0–10 numeric pain intensity scale

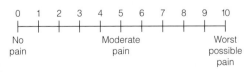

Brief word instructions[30]

For children, pictorial images are used. The nurse points to each face using the words to describe the pain intensity. The child chooses the face that best describes the pain they are experiencing. The number is then recorded.

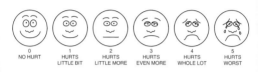

| 0 | 1 | 2 | 3 | 4 | 5 |
| NO HURT | HURTS LITTLE BIT | HURTS LITTLE MORE | HURTS EVEN MORE | HURTS WHOLE LOT | HURTS WORST |

■ COMMON SITES OF REFERRED PAIN FROM VARIOUS BODY ORGANS[31]

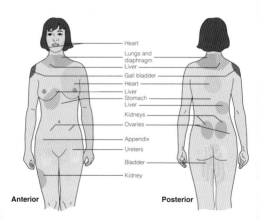

■ THE FOUR ABDOMINAL QUADRANTS[13]

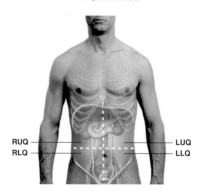

RUQ ——   —— LUQ
RLQ ——   —— LLQ

Organs in the four abdominal quadrants

RIGHT UPPER QUADRANT (RUQ)	LEFT UPPER QUADRANT (LUQ)
Liver	Stomach
Gallbladder	Spleen
Duodenum	Left lobe of liver
Head of pancreas	Body of pancreas
Right kidney and adrenal	Left kidney and adrenal
Hepatic flexure of colon	Splenic flexure of colon
Part of ascending and transverse colon	Part of transverse and descending colon

(Continued)

RIGHT LOWER QUADRANT (RLQ)	LEFT LOWER QUADRANT (LLQ)
Caecum	Part of descending colon
Appendix	Sigmoid colon
Right ovary and tube	Left ovary and tube
Right ureter	Left ureter
Right spermatic cord	Left spermatic cord

MIDLINE
Aorta
Uterus
Bladder

Blood values[32]

Atomic symbols

Ca	Calcium
C	Carbon
Cl	Chloride
H	Hydrogen
Mg	Magnesium
O	Oxygen
K	Potassium
Na	Sodium
PO	Phosphate
HCO_3	Bicarbonate

Cardiac enzymes

Note: These normal adult values are a typical range and are relative to the type of test, equipment used and weight of patient. They are a guide only.

MARKER	NORMAL LEVEL	ONSET	PEAKS	DURATION
Creatine kinase (CK)	M: 55–170 U/L F: 30–135 U/L	3–6 hours	12–24 hours	24–48 hours
Creatine kinase-muscle/blood (CK-MB)	<5% of total CK activity	4–8 hours	18–24 hours	72 hours
Troponin (cTn)	Variable depending on methodology	2–4 hours	24–36 hours	7–10 days

Electrolytes

Sodium (Na)	134–146 mmol/L
Potassium (K)	3.4–5.0 mmol/L
Chloride (Cl)	98–108 mmol/L
Bicarbonate (HCO_3)	22–29 mmol/L
Anion gap	8–16 mmol/L
Osmolality calculated	275–295 mmol/L
Glucose	3.0–7.8 mmol/L; 3.9–6.2 mmol/L (fasting)
Urea (age-dependent)	4.0–8.0 mmol/L
Creatinine	0.7–1.2 mg/dL for adult male (60 to 110 Micromoles per litre) 0.5–1.0 mg/dL for adult female (45 to 90 Micromoles per litre)
Protein total	63–78 g/L
Albumin	35–45 g/L
Globulin	25–45 g/L

Bilirubin total	3–17 mmol/L
Alkaline phosphatase (ALP) (age-dependent)	35–150 U/L
Gamma—GT (GGT)	5–40 U/L
Alanine transaminase (ALT)	1–45 U/L
Aspartate transaminase (AST)	1–36 U/L
Calcium (Ca)	2.15–2.60 mmol/L
Calcium (alb. Corr.)	2.15–2.60 mmol/L
Phosphate (PO)	0.80–1.40 mmol/L
Magnesium (Mg)	0.70–1.10 mmol/L
Triglycerides	<200 mg/dL; <2.0 mmol/L (fasting)
Low-density lipoprotein (LDL)	<80 mg/dL; 2.0–3.4 mmol/L (fasting)
High-density lipoprotein (HDL)	>35 mg/dL; 0.9–2.2 mmol/L (fasting)
Total cholesterol	<200 mg/dL; <5.5 mmol/L (fasting)

Note: Variations may occur depending on the age and sex of the patient.

Blood gases

pH	7.36–7.44
pCO_2	35–45 mm Hg
PaO_2	80–100 mm Hg
Bicarbonate (HCO_3)	22–29 mmol/L
Base excess (BE)	–3 to +3 mmol/L
Oxygen saturation (SaO_2)	94–98%

Thyroid function test

TSH	1–11 mU/L

Drug levels

Digoxin	toxic	>2 mg/L
	normal	1–2 mg/L
Paracetamol	toxic	30 mg/L
	normal	5–25 mg/L

Haematology

WBC age-related	4.5–11×10⁹/L
RBC age-related	Male: 4.6–6.2×10⁹/L
	Female: 4.2–5.4×10⁹/L
Hb	Male: 130–180 g/L
	Female: 120–160 g/L
Hct	Male: 45–54 mL/dL
	Female: 37–47 mL/dL
MCV	80–100 fL
Platelets	150–400×10⁹/L
Lymphocytes	25–33%
Monocytes	3–7%

Note: Variations may occur depending on the age and sex of the patient.

Normal values in a urinalysis

pH	4.6–8.0
Specific gravity (SG)	1.003–1.030
Protein	<0.15 g/day
Blood	up to 2 RBCs
Glucose	nil
Ketones	nil
Osmolality	38–1400 mOsm/kg H_2O

Mental health assessment

Mental health service users are usually referred to as consumers or clients. It is very important that you gather as much information as possible in your initial assessment. To do this, you need to quickly develop trust and rapport with the person. Be personable and genuine, and ask open-ended questions. This approach will elicit the most information. Gather information under the following broad headings:

Personal—identifying information

- Name
- Age
- Sexuality
- Gender
- Occupation
- Next of kin/Significant other
- Cultural affiliation
- Medications
- Previous treatment
- Physical illnesses
- What does the person see as the presenting problem? That is, what brought them in today?

Appearance—person's physical presentation (factual—do NOT use emotive adjectives as descriptors)

- Grooming
- Posture
- Make-up
- Hygiene
- Tattoos/Piercing
- Clothes
- Scars
- Other

Mood—variability, intensity and appropriateness

- Worried (about?)
- Tearful (cause?)
- Angry (with whom or what?)
- Elated
- Irritable
- Scared (of what?)
- Flat
- Hopeless
- Labile

Behaviour—behaviour exhibited/context

- Calm
- Tremors
- Facial movements
- Attitude
- Hyperactive
- Agitated (in what way?)
- Rigid
- Aggressive
- Gestures inappropriate/ appropriate
- Language/words used
- Suspicious

Perception—check the five senses (visual, auditory, tactile, olfactory, gustatory)

- Hallucinations (alterations in sensory perception)
- Illusions

Thoughts—processes and content observed in conversation

- Delusions (fixed false beliefs)
- Paranoia (who and what?)
- Concrete thoughts (regarding?)
- Thought blocking
- Phobias (what?)
- Tangential thoughts
- Obsessions (about?)
- Other

Safety—ask direct questions

- Suicide: Are you thinking of hurting yourself—How? When? Do you have a plan?
- Homicide: Is there someone you think you could harm? Who? How? When? Do you have a plan?

Risk—who might be at risk and from what?

People with a mental illness are often vulnerable. They might be the one who is at risk. Document in what ways. What other risks might there be (e.g. property, children, job, reputation, finances)?

Memory—brief cognitive assessment
- Orientation
- Concentration
- Alertness

Insight and judgement—person's awareness about condition and decision making
- Ask client about the nature of the illness. Is self-assessment realistic/unrealistic?
- Ask questions like, 'What would you do if you saw an old lady lying on the road?'
- Explore the client's impulse control.

Check information with relatives and other staff who may know the person. Avoid being confrontational; give the person an explanation as to what you are doing. Be aware of your own biases, attitudes and judgemental behaviour, and how you present to the client. Write up notes in an objective, professional manner, noting the context of assessment and persons present.

Resuscitation

■ **CARDIAC RHYTHMS**[33]

Sinus rhythm
Sinus rhythm is the normal rhythm of the heart and consists of the following wave formations.

P wave	represents contraction of the atria.
PR interval	should be no greater than 0.2 seconds or 5 small squares.

QRS complex represents contraction of the ventricles and should be no wider than 0.12 seconds or 3 small squares.

T wave is the resting phase of the heart.

Electrocardiogram (ECG) paper
- Time is measured on the horizontal axis.
- Voltage is measured on the vertical axis.
- Each small square = 0.04 seconds.
- 1 large square (5 small squares) = 0.2 seconds.

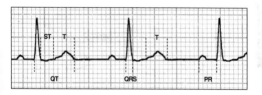

To calculate rate
Count the number of large squares between two R waves and divide 300 by this number.

Location of the anterior ribs, the angle of Louis and placement of chest leads (V leads) for a 12-lead electrocardiogram

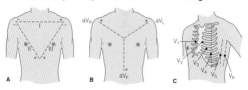

Usual waveform of an ECG

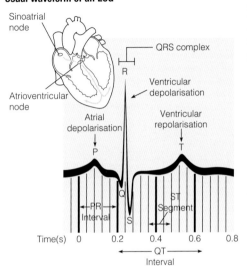

To work out the rate:

1. Count 30 large boxes.
2. Count the number of R waves within the 30 boxes—
   i.e. 7 in this example.
3. Multiply the number of R waves by 10—i.e. 7 × 10 = rate
   70 beats/min.

■ WHEN TO SEEK HELP/PATIENT REVIEW

AREA	SIGNS AND SYMPTOMS FOR ADULTS
AIRWAY	Threatened airway (i.e. person having difficulty breathing or noisy breathing)
BREATHING	• Use of accessory muscles or sternal recession • Respiratory rate <12 or >25 breaths/minute • SpO$_2$ of less than 95% • Respiratory arrest
CIRCULATION	• A change in HR of 20 beats/minute from the patient's baseline parameters, or a pulse rate <50 or >120 beats/minute • A change in BP of 20 mm Hg from the patient's baseline parameters or a systolic blood pressure <90 mm Hg • Cardiac arrest
NEUROLOGICAL	• Sudden fall in consciousness or difficult to arouse • Fall in the Glasgow Coma Scale of >2 points • Seizures
OTHER	• Any person you are concerned about

ALWAYS SEEK HELP SOONER RATHER THAN LATER.

■ CPR[25]

CPR for cardiopulmonary resuscitation

	AIRWAY	COMPRESSION	
			1 or 2 people
Infants <1 year	Chin lift or jaw thrust only—no head tilt	2 fingers	30:2
Younger child: 1–8 years	Chin lift or jaw thrust; head tilt more than infants but less than adults	Heel of one hand	30:2
Older child: 9–14 years	Chin lift, jaw thrust or head tilt	2 hands	30:2
Adult	Chin lift, jaw thrust or head tilt	2 hands	30:2

■ BASIC LIFE SUPPORT FLOW CHART

Basic Life Support

D — **Dangers?**

R — **Responsive?**

S — **Send** for help

A — Open **Airway**

B — Normal **Breathing?**

C — Start **CPR**
30 compressions : 2 breaths

D — Attach **Defibrillator (AED)**
as soon as available, follow prompts

Continue CPR until responsiveness or normal breathing return

January 2016

NEW ZEALAND
Resuscitation Council
WHAKAHAUORA AOTEAROA

■ PAEDIATRIC ADVANCED CARDIOVASCULAR LIFE SUPPORT

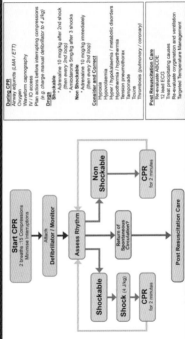

Advanced Life Support for Infants and Children

During CPR
- Airway adjuncts (LMA / ETT)
- Oxygen
- Waveform capnography
- IV / IO access
- Plan actions before interrupting compressions (e.g. charge manual defibrillator to 4 J/kg)

Drugs
Shockable
- Adrenaline 10 mcg/kg after 2nd shock (then every 2nd loop)
- Amiodarone 5mg/kg after 3 shocks
Non Shockable
- Adrenaline 10 mcg/kg immediately (then every 2nd loop)

Consider and Correct
- Hypoxia
- Hypovolaemia
- Hyper / hypokalaemia / metabolic disorders
- Hypothermia / hyperthermia
- Tension pneumothorax
- Tamponade
- Toxins
- Thrombosis (pulmonary / coronary)

Post Resuscitation Care
- Re-evaluate ABCDE
- 12 lead ECG
- Treat precipitating causes
- Re-evaluate oxygenation and ventilation
- Targeted Temperature Management

NEW ZEALAND
Resuscitation Council
WHAKAORA AOTEAROA

Start CPR
2 breaths : 15 Compressions
Minimise interruptions

Attach Defibrillator / Monitor

Assess Rhythm

Shockable → **Shock (4 J/kg)** → **CPR** for 2 minutes

Non Shockable → **CPR** for 2 minutes

Return of Spontaneous Circulation?

Post Resuscitation Care

January 2016

■ ADULT ADVANCED CARDIOVASCULAR LIFE SUPPORT

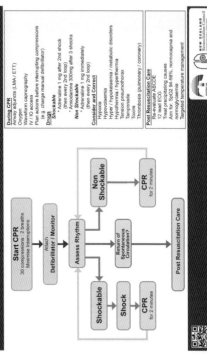

Advanced Life Support for Adults

Start CPR
30 compressions : 2 breaths
Minimise interruptions

Attach Defibrillator / Monitor

Assess Rhythm

Shockable → **Shock** → **CPR for 2 minutes**

Non Shockable → **CPR for 2 minutes**

Return of Spontaneous Circulation?

Post Resuscitation Care

During CPR
Airway adjuncts (LMA / ETT)
Oxygen
Waveform capnography
IV / IO access
Plan actions before interrupting compressions
(e.g. charge manual defibrillator)

Drugs
Shockable
• Adrenaline 1 mg after 2nd shock
(then every 2nd loop)
• Amiodarone 300mg after 3 shocks
Non Shockable
• Adrenaline 1 mg immediately
(then every 2nd loop)

Consider and Correct
Hypoxia
Hypovolaemia
Hyper / hypokalaemia / metabolic disorders
Hypothermia / hyperthermia
Tension pneumothorax
Tamponade
Toxins
Thrombosis (pulmonary / coronary)

Post Resuscitation Care
Re-evaluate ABCDE
12 lead ECG
Treat precipitating causes
Aim for SpO2 94-98%, normocapnia and normoglycaemia
Targeted temperature management

January 2016

■ CHOKING FLOW CHART

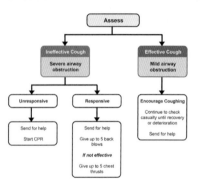

Foreign Body Airway Obstruction (Choking)

Assess

Ineffective Cough — Severe airway obstruction

Effective Cough — Mild airway obstruction

Unresponsive
- Send for help
- Start CPR

Responsive
- Send for help
- Give up to 5 back blows
- *If not effective*
- Give up to 5 chest thrusts

Encourage Coughing
- Continue to check casualty until recovery or deterioration
- Send for help

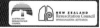

NEW ZEALAND
Resuscitation Council
WHAKAHAUORA AOTEAROA

Wound care

■ FACTORS THAT INHIBIT HEALING[34]

GENERAL FACTORS	LOCAL FACTORS
• Developmental considerations • Age • Underlying disease • Vascularity • Nutritional status • Obesity • Disorders of sensation/ movement • Medications • Psychological state • Radiation therapy • Lifestyle	• Wound management practices • Hydration of wound • Temperature of wound • Pressure, friction, shearing forces • Foreign bodies • Infection

■ WOUND TYPES[35]

TYPE	CAUSE	DESCRIPTION AND CHARACTERISTICS
Incision	Sharp instrument (e.g. knife or scalpel)	Open wound; deep or shallow
Contusion	Blow from a blunt instrument	Closed wound; skin appears ecchymotic (bruised) because of damaged blood vessels

(Continued)

Abrasion	Surface scrape, either unintentional (e.g. scraped knee from a fall) or intentional (e.g. dermal abrasion to remove pockmarks)	Open wound involving the skin
Puncture	Penetration of the skin and often the underlying tissues by a sharp instrument, either intentional or unintentional	Open wound
Laceration	Tissues torn apart, often from accidents (e.g. with machinery)	Open wound; edges are often jagged
Penetrating wound	Penetration of the skin and the underlying tissues, usually unintentional (e.g. from a bullet or metal fragments)	Open wound

■ PHASES OF WOUND HEALING[35]

Inflammatory phase: occurs immediately after injury, lasting 3–6 days.
Proliferative phase: extends from day 3–4 to about day 21.
Maturation phase: begins about day 21 and can extend 1–2 years after injury.

■ WOUND ASSESSMENT[34]

Effective wound management requires the nurse to assess:
- the patient
- the wound (remember: 'WE ASSESS').

The patient ◄────► The wound

Identify factors that inhibit healing:
- nutritional status
- medications
- adjunct therapy
- weight for height
- mobility

- Ⓦound type and healing
- Ⓔxudate—amount; colour/type; odour/consistency
- Ⓐppearance (see below)
- Ⓢize/Location/Width/Length/Depth
- Ⓢurrounding skin and signs of infection
- Ⓔdges
- Ⓢcale of tissue loss
- Ⓢtated pain

Appearance

COLOUR	POTENTIAL MEANING	ACTION
Pink	Epithelialising	Protect
Red	Granulating	Protect
Yellow	Sloughy	Clean
Green	Infected	Clean
Black	Necrotic	Debride

Wound exudate

TYPE	DESCRIPTION
Serous	Clear, straw-coloured fluid
Haemoserous	Blood-stained; serous fluid
Sanguineous	Frank or heavily blood-stained
Purulent	Contains pus

Signs of infection

WOUND	SYSTEMIC
• Pain	• Elevated temperature
• Heat	• Malaise
• Oedema	• Raised leucocyte count
• Erythema	• Sepsis
• Exudate	

Classification of wounds for infection

Clean	• Made under aseptic surgical conditions • Do not enter genitourinary or respiratory tracts, or alimentary tract/oropharyngeal cavity • No signs of infection

Clean/ Contaminated	• Wounds entering abovementioned tracts/cavities • Contaminated by resident flora of cavities but no host reaction
Contaminated	• Contaminated by bacteria causing host reaction but no pus
Infected	• Clinical signs of infection present • Increased leucocyte/macrophage levels

■ PRESSURE INJURIES

A pressure injury can be defined as 'a localised injury to the skin and/or underlying tissue usually over bony prominences as a result of pressure, or shear and/or friction, or a combination of these factors'.[36]

■ STAGES OF PRESSURE INJURIES[35, 36]

Stage I Pressure injury
Non-blanching erythema

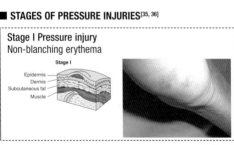

Stage I

Epidermis
Dermis
Subcutaneous fat
Muscle

(Continued)

Stage II Pressure injury
Partial-thickness skin loss involving epidermis and possibly dermis

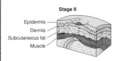

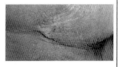

Stage III Pressure injury
Full-thickness skin loss involving subcutaneous tissue that may extend to, but not through, underlying fascia

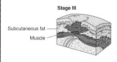

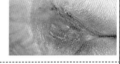

Stage IV Pressure injury
Full-thickness skin loss involving muscle, bone or supporting structures

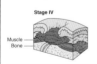

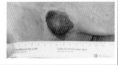

Unstageable/unclassified
Pressure injury: depth unknown

 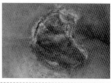

Suspected deep tissue injury
Depth unknown

 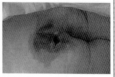

PRESSURE INJURY RISK ASSESSMENT TOOLS[37]

The ACSQHC advises that, to prevent or minimise harm, clinicians should utilise effective screening tools designed to identify patients at risk of developing pressure injuries.[11]

WATERLOW PRESSURE INJURY RISK ASSESSMENT SCALE

Build/weight for height		Skin type and visual risk areas		Sex and age		Special risks: tissue malnutrition	
Average	0	Healthy	0	Male	1	e.g. Terminal cachexia	8
Above average	1	Tissue paper	1	Female	2	Cardiac failure	5
Obese	2	Dry	1	14–49	1	Periph vascular disease	5
Below average	3	Oedematous	1	50–64	2	Anaemia	2
		Clammy (temp)	1	65–74	3	Smoking	1
Continence		Discoloured	2	75–80	4		
Complete/catheterised	0	Broken/spot	3	81+	5	**Neurological deficit**	
Occasion incont	1					e.g. Diabetes, MS, CVA,	
Cath/incontinent of faeces	2	**Mobility**		**Appetite**		Motor/sensory	
Doubly incont	3	Fully	0	Average	0	paraplegia	4–6
		Restless/fidgety	1	Poor	1		
		Apathetic	2	NG tube/fluids only	2	**Major surgery/trauma**	
		Restricted	3	NBM/anorexic	3	Orthopaedic	
		Inert/traction	4			Below waist, spinal	5
		Chair-bound	5			On table >2 hours	5
						Medication	
						Cytotoxics	
						High-dose steroids, anti-	
						inflammatory	4

Score: 10+ at risk; 15+ high risk; 20+ very high risk

■ PRESSURE INJURY PREVENTION

- Identify and eliminate cause.
- Educate—risk and prevention.
- Increase activity/mobilisation.
- Avoid smoking.
- Promote healthy nutrition.
- Protect skin—cleanse, moisturise, maintain pH.
- Manage incontinence.
- Implement repositioning regimens.
- Check support surfaces.
- Use protective devices.
- Use appropriate transfer equipment.

WOUND-CARE PRODUCTS

PRODUCT	ACTION	TYPE OF WOUND
FOAM	• Absorbs, insulates • Promotes autolysis of devitalised tissue	• Needing absorption • Needing protection ***Note:*** *Not highly exudating*
HYDROGELS	• Retains moisture, rehydrates • Promotes autolysis of devitalised tissue • Cools surface of wound • Is oxygen permeable	• Needing hydration • Needing autolysis ***Note:*** *Not highly exudating*
ALGINATES	• Forms hydrophilic gel when in contact with wound exudate • Facilitates debridement and rehydration of dead tissue	• Cavities • Sinuses • Infected • Needing debridement ***Note:*** *Not dry wounds*
TRANSPARENT FILMS	• Promotes epithelialisation • Creates moist environment • Protects from friction	• Needing protection • Needing hydration ***Note:*** *Not exudating; caution fragile skin*

PRODUCT	ACTION	TYPE OF WOUND
HYDRO FIBRE	• Made of non-woven sodium carbo-xymethylcellulose spun into fibres • Converts to gel on contact with exudate • Wicking of exudate • More absorbent than alginates	• Infected wounds • Needing absorption
CADEXOMER IODINE-MEDICATED DRESSINGS	• Composed of a three-dimensional starch lattice formed into spherical microbeads with 0.9% iodine • Cadexomer base absorbs exudate, swells, then forms gel	• Heavily exudating • Needing desloughing • Needing antimicrobial effect
	Note: Not for patients who are sensitive to iodine, those with thyroid disorders, pregnant or lactating women, children aged 2 or younger, or those with large wounds. Should not exceed 3 months in a single course of treatment	

(Continued)

PRODUCT	ACTION	TYPE OF WOUND
SILICONE	• Gentle adhesive and removal properties • Minimises wound trauma on removal • Conforms to different anatomical shapes	• Needing protection *Note: Not for patients with allergy to silicone products*
HYDROCOLLOIDS	• Polymers interact with wound exudate and become gelatinous mass • Protects wounds • Maintains moisture • Waterproof barrier • Promotes autolysis of devitalised tissue	• Needing protection • Needing hydration • Needing autolysis *Note: Not infected; not involving bone*
SILVERS	• Converts into an ionic form to produce antimicrobial effect • Antimicrobial efficacy of dressing determined by the concentration of silver—needs moisture for silver to be released	• Moderate to heavily exudating • Colonised *Note: Should be used prudently*

■ CALCULATION OF ANKLE/BRACHIAL PRESSURE INDEX (ABPI)[38]

The ankle/brachial pressure index is a Doppler measurement which helps to determine the degree of arterial or venous disease in the leg.

To calculate the ABPI, divide the highest ankle systolic pressure in each leg by the highest brachial reading in both arms:

$$\frac{\text{Ankle systolic pressure}}{\text{Brachial systolic pressure}} = \text{ABPI}$$

Normal	>0.9
Claudiant	0.5–1
Ischaemic	<0.5
Calcified	>1.2

Ankle/brachial pressure index

<0.5	0.5–0.7	0.7–0.8
Arterial ulcer	Mixed arterial–venous ulcer	
>0.8–1.2	>1.2	
Venous ulcer	Possible calcified vessels	

■ SKIN TEARS

The STAR skin tear classification system[39]

Category 1a
A skin tear where the edges **can** be realigned to the normal anatomical position (without undue stretching) and the skin or flap colour **is not** pale, dusky or darkened.

Category 1b
A skin tear where the edges **can** be realigned to the normal anatomical position (without undue stretching) and the skin or flap colour **is** pale, dusky or darkened.

Category 2a
A skin tear where the edges **cannot** be realigned to the normal anatomical position and the skin or flap colour **is not** pale, dusky or darkened.

Category 2b
A skin tear where the edges **cannot** be realigned to the normal anatomical position and the skin or flap colour **is** pale, dusky or darkened.

Category 3
A skin tear where the skin flap is completely absent.

Skin tear prevention[34, 35]

- Assess for falls risk and implement prevention strategies.
- Use gentle and timely handling on transfer and repositioning.
- Use devices that reduce shear and friction.

- Cover vulnerable skin surfaces with protective clothing or devices.
- Maintain position with pillows and foam wedges to prevent shear. (Satin or silk covers will further reduce shear forces.)
- Moisturise the skin frequently to reduce dryness.
- Avoid perfumed soaps that dry and alter the skin's pH.
- Cease smoking.
- Maintain adequate hydration and optimal nutrition.
- Avoid adhesive tapes and dressings on fragile skin in favour of roller or tubular bandages.
- Review medications and eliminate, if possible, those that alter the skin's integrity.
- Control any co-morbidities that alter the skin's condition or risk of injury.
- Provide patient and carer education on skin health and injury prevention.

Nursing process[40]

The nursing process provides a framework for organising nursing care.

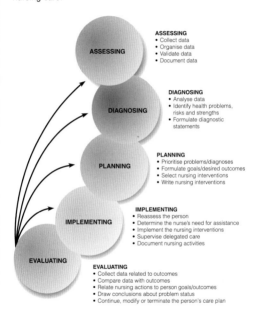

ASSESSING
- Collect data
- Organise data
- Validate data
- Document data

DIAGNOSING
- Analyse data
- Identify health problems, risks and strengths
- Formulate diagnostic statements

PLANNING
- Prioritise problems/diagnoses
- Formulate goals/desired outcomes
- Select nursing interventions
- Write nursing interventions

IMPLEMENTING
- Reassess the person
- Determine the nurse's need for assistance
- Implement the nursing interventions
- Supervise delegated care
- Document nursing activities

EVALUATING
- Collect data related to outcomes
- Compare data with outcomes
- Relate nursing actions to person goals/outcomes
- Draw conclusions about problem status
- Continue, modify or terminate the person's care plan

■ CLINICAL REASONING CYCLE[41]

A nurse's clinical reasoning ability is intrinsic to the delivery of quality care. The clinical reasoning cycle outlined below provides nurses with a framework to follow in order to develop and hone their clinical reasoning ability.

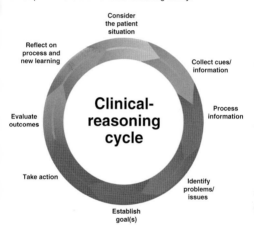

Documentation[42]

The ACSQHC highlights the importance of effective communication, reminding clinicians that communication is inherent to patient care. It is therefore critical that effective systems and processes are utilised to facilitate optimal communication and documentation methods at all times.

■ PRACTICE GUIDELINES FOR ALL DOCUMENTATION (WRITTEN OR ELECTRONIC)[43]

Do

- Chart a change in a patient's condition and show that follow-up actions were taken.
- Read the nurses' notes prior to care to determine if there has been a change in the patient's condition.
- Be timely. A late entry is better than no entry; however, the longer the period of time between actual care and charting, the greater the suspicion.
- Use objective, specific and factual descriptions.
- Correct charting for errors.
- Chart all teaching.
- Record the patient's actual words by putting quotation marks around the words.
- Chart the patient's response to interventions.
- Review your notes. Are they clear and do they reflect what you want to say?

Don't

- Leave a blank space for a colleague to chart later.
- Chart in advance of the event (e.g. procedure, medication).
- Use vague terms (e.g. 'appears to be comfortable', 'had a good night').
- Chart for someone else.
- Use 'patient' or 'client', as it is their chart.
- Alter a record even if requested by a superior or a doctor.
- Record assumptions or words reflecting bias (e.g. 'complainer', 'disagreeable').

■ WRITING WITH SOAPIE[43]

S = Subjective	What the patient/significant other verbalises
O = Objective	Data that is measured and observed
A = Assessment	What is diagnosed from the data gathered
P = Planning	What care has been planned
I = Implementation	What care has been implemented
E = Evaluation	What the outcomes are

Writing with PIE

P = Problem
I = Implementation
E = Evaluation

Clinical handover

■ ISBAR[44]

Clinical handover checklist	
I Identification	• Introductions—patients and transitioning staff • ID band present on patient • ID band details correct • Oxygen and suction check at bedside
S Situation	• Current diagnosis and immediate concern • Alerts/allergies • Infectious status (contact, airborne, droplet)

(Continued)

B Background	• Relevant patient history and symptoms • Planned care and interventions • Examination results
A Assessment	• Review vital signs and score • Review fluid balance record and fluid orders • Check current treatment—med chart, IV infusions, NGT and any other therapy • Check invasive devices—cannula, tubes, drains • Review ADLs and status of falls and pressure injury risk • Safety check—5Bs (see page 17)
R Recommendation	• Upcoming procedures/treatments/further action • Investigation required • Discharge plan • Questions

■ PACE

A valuable aspect of communicating in stressful situations is a learned skill called graded assertiveness. This skill aids the clinician to communicate, advocate and direct others in high-stress environments. One method of employing graded assertiveness is referred to as PACE.

PROBE—'Did you know that this patient has an allergy to penicillin?'

ALERT—'I think that medication you are about to give contains penicillin. Let's check it again.'

CHALLENGE—'It risks patient safety and is against our policy to administer medication that a patient is allergic to. You should not continue.'

EMERGENCY—'Step away from the patient. You will not administer this medication. I am contacting my team leader immediately.'

Time management grid

To organise your day, you may choose to use a time management grid as set out on the following page.

PATIENT NAME AND BED NUMBER	WHAT IS DUE TIME IN HOURS									
	0700	0800	0900	1000	1100	1200	1300	1400	1500
Mr Jones 1		meds	PAC	obs	PAC	xray	PAC	obs	PAC
Mr Smith 2	shower	CT	walk A2	meds		assist meal		obs	
Mrs Wills 3	IV check	IV check meds	IV check	IV check obs	IV check	IV check meds	IV check	IV check obs	FBC IV check
Mr Davis 4	shower obs	obs	obs	meds obs	obs	obs	obs	obs	obs

CODES:

obs:	observation
CT:	cat scan
PAC:	pressure area scan
walk A2:	walk assist × 2 persons
IV check:	site check, infusion check, fluid balance chart record
FBC:	fluid balance chart tally

The National Safety and Quality Health Service (NSQHS) Standards[1]

To improve the quality of patient care and promote patient safety, the ACSQHC developed the National Safety and Quality Health Service (NSQHS) Standards. The Standards prioritise key areas of safety and quality where it is known that patients experience higher levels of harm, and where there is good evidence that improved care could result in better patient outcomes. Standards include:

- Clinical Governance for Health Service Organisations
- Partnering with Consumers
- Preventing and Controlling Healthcare-associated Infection
- Medication Safety
- Comprehensive Care
- Communicating for Safety
- Blood Management
- Recognising and Responding to Acute Deterioration

General abbreviations

Note: *Any abbreviations used should be accepted within your health care organisation prior to use.*

| ABG | arterial blood gas |
| ADL | activities of daily living |

AMI	acute myocardial infarction
ARDS	acute respiratory distress syndrome
bd	12-hourly/twice a day
BO	bowels open
Bx	biopsy
Ca	cancer
CAD	coronary artery disease
CCF	congestive cardiac failure
CHD	congenital heart disease
CHF	congestive heart failure
COAD	chronic obstructive airways disease
COPD	chronic obstructive pulmonary disease
CPR	cardio pulmonary resuscitation
CVA	cerebral vascular accident
CVP	central venous pressure
CWMS	colour, warmth, movement, sensation
CXR	chest X-ray
d	day
D	dose
DOB	date of birth
ECG	electrocardiogram
FBC	full blood count
FUO	fever of unknown origin
HACC	home and community care
HNPU	has not passed urine
HR	heart rate
Hx	history
ICC	intercostal catheter
IDC	indwelling catheter
IHD	ischaemic heart disease
IVC	intravenous catheter/cannula

IVT	intravenous therapy
JVP	jugular venous pressure
LFT	liver function test
MCS	microscopic culture sensitivity
MI	myocardial infarction
MRSA	multiple/methicillin-resistant *staphylococcus aureus*
MSA	mental state assessment
MSE	mental state examination
MSU	mid-stream urine
MVA	motor vehicle accident
NAD	nil abnormalities detected
NBM	nil by mouth
NGT	nasogastric tube
NIDDM	non-insulin-dependent diabetes mellitus (better to use Type 2 DM)
NKA	no known allergies
NOF	neck of femur
O_2	oxygen
Obs	observation
OE	on examination
OR	operating room
ORIF	open reduction and internal fixation
OT	occupational therapy/operating theatre
PAC	pressure area care
PCA	patient-controlled analgesia
PD	patient diagnosis/peritoneal dialysis/provisional diagnosis
PE	physical examination/pulmonary embolus
PEG	percutaneous endoscopic gastronomy tube
PICC	peripherally inserted central catheter

PND	paroxysmal nocturnal dyspnoea/postnatal depression
POP	plaster of Paris
PU	passed urine
PUO	pyrexia unknown origin
PVD	peripheral vascular disease
RLL	right lower lobe
RO	removal of
ROM	range of motion
RR	respiratory rate
SI	international system of units
SOB	shortness of breath
SSRI	selective serotonin reuptake inhibitor
Staph	staphylococcus
TAH	total abdominal hysterectomy
TIA	transient ischaemic attack
TPN	total parenteral nutrition
TPR	temperature, pulse, respiration
Tx	treatment
UA	urinalysis
UR	**unique** record
URTI	upper respiratory tract infection
UTI	urinary tract infection
UWSD	underwater sealed drainage
VTE	venous thromboembolism
WBC	white blood cell
Wt	weight
yo	years old

Useful websites

----

www.acccn.com.au
Australian College of Critical Care Nurses

www.midwives.org.au
Australian College of Midwives

www.acn.edu.au
Australian College of Nursing

www.ahpra.gov.au
Australian Health Practitioner Regulation Agency

www.anmf.org.au
Australian Nursing & Midwifery Federation

www.anmac.org.au
Australian Nursing & Midwifery Accreditation Council
(ANMAC)

www.resus.org.au
Australian Resuscitation Council

www.cochrane.org
Cochrane

www.catsinam.org.au
Congress of Aboriginal and Torres Strait Islander Nurses and
Midwives (CATSINaM)

www.joannabriggs.org
Joanna Briggs Institute

www.nhmrc.gov.au
National Health and Medical Research Council

www.woundsaustralia.com.au
WoundsAustralia

Endnotes

1. Australian Commission on Safety and Quality in Health Care (2017). *National Safety and Quality Health Service Standards.* Sydney: ACSQHC.

2. National Health and Medical Research Council (2010). *Clinical educators guide for the prevention and control of infection in healthcare.*

3. Australian Commission on Safety and Quality in Health Care (2017). *Preventing and Controlling Healthcare-Associated Infection Standard.* Sydney: ACSQHC.

4. National Health and Medical Research Council (2010). *Australian guidelines for the prevention and control of infection in healthcare.* Retrieved from: <https://www.nhmrc.gov.au/guidelines-publications/cd33>

5. Workplace Health and Safety Queensland (2017). *Guide for handling cytotixic drugs and related waste.* O.o.I. Relations, Editor. Retrieved from <https://www.worksafe.qld.gov.au>

6. World Health Organization [WHO] (2018). *5 moments for handy hygiene.* Retrieved from: <http://www.who.int/gpsc/5may/background/5moments/en>

7. Hales, M. (2018). Infection prevention and control. In A. Berman, S. Snyder, G. Frandsen, T. Levett-Jones, T. Dwyer, M. Hales … D. Stanley (Eds), *Kozier & Erb's fundamentals of nursing* Vol. 2 (4th ed.). Melbourne, Vic.: Pearson Australia.

8. Department of Health (2017). *Management of occupational exposure to blood and body fluids.* Retrieved from <https://www.health.qld.gov.au/__data/assets/pdf_file/0016/151162/qh-gdl-321-8.pdf>

9. Queensland Health (2010). *Patient handling: Better practice guidelines* (2nd ed.) (Part A: 33-36). Brisbane, Qld: Queensland Health.

10. Australian Commission on Safety and Quality in Health Care (2009). *Preventing falls and harm from falls in older*

people: Best practice guidelines for Australian community care. Sydney: ACSQHC.

11.   Australian Commission on Safety and Quality in Health Care (2017). *Comprehensive Care Standard*. Sydney: ACSQHC.

12.   Australian Commission on Safety and Quality in Health Care (2009). *Preventing falls and harm from falls in older people: best practice guidelines for Australian hospitals*. Sydney: ACSQHC.

13.   Nicol, M., Bavin, C., Cronin, P., Rawlings-Anderson, K., Cole, E., & Hunter, J. (2012). *Essential Nursing Skills E-Book*, p. 53. Elsevier Health Sciences.

14.   Corwin, M. (2018). Sudden infant death syndrome: risk factors and risk reduction strategies. *UpTo Date*, June 21.

15.   Australian Commission on Safety and Quality in Health Care (2017). *Medication Safety Standard*. Sydney: ACSQHC.

16.   Australian Commission on Safety and Quality in Health Care (2009). *Guidelines for use of the National Inpatient Medication Chart, including paediatric version*. Sydney: ACSQHC.

17.   Queensland Government (Ed.) (2015). *Peripheral intravenous catheter (PIVC): maintenance*. Queensland: Department of Health.

18.   Australian Commission on Safety and Quality in Health Care (2017). *APINCHS Classification of High Risk Medicines*. Sydney: ACSQHC.

19.   Bryant, B. & Knights, K. (2014). *Pharmacology for health professionals ebook* (4th ed.). Sydney: Elsevier Australia.

20.   O'Driscoll, B. R., et. al. (2017). BTS guideline for oxygen use in adults in healthcare and emergency settings, *Thorax, 72*(1), doi:10.1136.

21.   Schrier, R. W. (2017). *Renal and electrolyte disorders* (8th ed.). Lippincott Williams & Wilkins.

22.   National Institute for Clinical Excellence (NICE) (2013). *Intravenous fluid therapy in adults in hospital*. NICE Guidance, CG174.

23. Royal Children's Hospital (2018). *Clinical practice guideline on intravenous fluids.* Retrieved from <http://www.rch.org.au/clinicalguide/index.cfm>

24. Australian Commission on Safety and Quality in Health Care (2017). *Recognising and Responding to Acute Deterioration Standard.* Sydney: ACSQHC.

25. Fleegler, E. & Kleinman, M. (2018). Pediatric advanced life support (PALS). *UpToDate*, June 13.

26. Teasdale, G., et al. (2014). The Glasgow Coma Scale at 40 years: standing the test of time. *The Lancet Neurology, 13*(8), 844–854.

27. Forbes, H. & Watt, E. (Eds) (2015). Assessing respiratory function. In C. Jarvis, *Jarvis's Physical examination and health assessment* (2nd ed.). Sydney: Elsevier Australia.

28. Walker, S. (2018). Fluid, electrolyte and acid-base balance. In A. Berman, S. Snyder, G. Frandsen, T. Levett-Jones, T. Dwyer, M. Hales … D. Stanley (Eds), *Kozier & Erb's fundamentals of nursing* Vol. 3 (4th ed.). Melbourne, Vic.: Pearson Australia.

29. Australian Resuscitation Council and New Zealand Resuscitation Council (2016). *Stroke: Guideline 9.2.2.* Retrieved from <https://www.nzrc.org.nz/assets/Guidelines/First-Aid/ANZCOR-Guideline-9-2-2-Stroke-Sep16.pdf>

30. Hockenberry, M. J., Wilson, D. & Rodgers, C. C. (Eds) (2017). *Wong's Essentials of Pediatric Nursing-E-Book* (10th ed.). Missouri: Elsevier.

31. Applegarth, J. & Flenady, T. (2018). Pain Management. In A. Berman, S. Snyder, G. Frandsen, T. Levett-Jones, T. Dwyer, M. Hales … D. Stanley (Eds), *Kozier & Erb's fundamentals of nursing* Vol. 3 (4th ed.). Melbourne, Vic.: Pearson Australia.

32. McCance, K. L. & Huether, S. E. (2015). *Pathophysiology: The biologic basis for disease in adults and children.* (7th ed.). London: Elsevier Health Sciences.

33. Goldberger, A. (2017). ECG tutorial: Rhythms and arrythmias of the sinus node. *UpTo Date*, July 3.

34. Carville, K. (2012). *Wound Care Manual* (6th ed.). Perth, Australia: Silver Chain Foundation.

35. Jans, C. (2018). Skin integrity and wound care. In A. Berman, S. Snyder, G. Frandsen, T. Levett-Jones, T. Dwyer, M. Hales … D. Stanley (Eds), *Kozier & Erb's fundamentals of nursing* Vol. 2 (4th ed.). Melbourne, Vic.: Pearson Australia.

36. Australian Wound Management Association (2012). *Pan Pacific clinical practice guideline for the prevention and management of pressure injury*. Osborne Park, WA: Cambridge Media.

37. Queensland Health, Health Service and Clinical Innovation Division (Ed.) (2014). *Pressure injury audit tools definitions*. Brisbane, Australia: Queensland Health.

38. Dwyer, T. & Friel, D. (2018). Circulation. In A. Berman, S. Snyder, G. Frandsen, T. Levett-Jones, T. Dwyer, M. Hales … D. Stanley (Eds), *Kozier & Erb's fundamentals of nursing* Vol. 3 (4th ed.). Melbourne, Vic.: Pearson Australia.

39. Carville, K., et al. (2007). STAR: A consensus for skin tear classification. *Primary Intention*, 2007. 15(1), 18–28.

40. Luxford, Y. (2018). Assessing. In A. Berman, S. Snyder, G. Frandsen, T. Levett-Jones, T. Dwyer, M. Hales … D. Stanley (Eds), *Kozier & Erb's fundamentals of nursing* Vol. 1 (4th ed.). Melbourne, Vic.: Pearson Australia.

41. Australian Commission on Safety and Quality in Health Care (2017). *Communicating for Safety Standard* (2nd ed.). Sydney: ACSQHC.

42. Courtney-Pratt, H. (2018). Documenting and Reporting. In A. Berman, S. Snyder, G. Frandsen, T. Levett-Jones, T. Dwyer, M. Hales … D. Stanley (Eds), *Kozier & Erb's fundamentals of nursing* Vol. 1 (4th ed.). Melbourne, Vic.: Pearson Australia.

43. Levett-Jones, T. (2018) Communicating. In A. Berman, S. Snyder, G. Frandsen, T. Levett-Jones, T. Dwyer, M. Hales …

D. Stanley (Eds), *Kozier & Erb's fundamentals of nursing* Vol. 2 (4th ed.). Melbourne, Vic.: Pearson Australia.

44. Zwaresnstein, M., Reeves,S. & Perrier,L.(2005). Effectiveness of Pre-licensure Interprofessional Education and Post-licensure Collaboartive Intervention. *Journal of Interprofessional Care, 19*, p. 148–165 and Adapted from Mikos, K (2007). In Berman, A.J., Snyder, S., Levett-Jones, T., Dwyer,T., Hales, M., Harvey, N ..., (2012). *Kozier and Erb's Fundamentals of Nursing*, Vol. 2, (2nd Aust. Ed) (p. 549). Sydney, NSW: Pearson Australia.

Credits

----

p. 40, Adapted with permission, from resources at The Royal Children's Hospital, Melbourne, Australia <https://www.rch.org. au/clinicalguide>; pp.42–43, Queensland Health. Queensland – Adult Deterioration Detection System (Q-ADDS). 2015. Central Queensland Hospital and Health Service (CQHHS), Rockhampton Hospital; p.48, Australian Resuscitation Council and New Zealand Resuscitation Council (ARC NRC) 2010, *Stroke: Guideline 9.2.2*, Australian Resuscitation Council and New Zealand Resuscitation Council, <http://www.resus.org.au>; p. 49 (middle), Adapted from Jarvis, C., *Physical examination and health assessment* (p. 167). 2015: Elsevier Health Sciences; p. 49 (bottom), Adapted from Heyer, E. J., Sharma, R., Winfree, C. J., Mocco, J., McMahon, D. J., McCormick, P. A., … Connolly, E. S. (2000). Severe Pain Confounds Neuropsychological Test Performance. Journal of Clinical and Experimental Neuropsychology, 22(5), 633–639. Reprinted by permission of the publisher (Taylor & Francis Ltd, http://www.tandfonline.com); p. 50 (top), © 1983 Wong-Baker FACES Foundation. <www.WongBakerFACES.org> Used with permission.; p. 50 (bottom), Berman, A. J., Snyder, S., Kozier, B. J., Erb, G., *Kozier & Erb's fundamentals of nursing*, 8th, © 2008. Printed by permission of Pearson Education, Inc., Upper Saddle River, New Jersey. p. 1134, figure 44.1; p. 60, Adapted from LeMone et al. (2011), p. 969; pp. 63–66, © The Australian Resuscitation Council; p. 69 & 79, Carville, K. (2012). *Wound care manual* (6th ed.). Osborne Park, WA: Silver Chain Foundation; p. 86, Sian Bradfield, Pearson Australia; p. 83, Adapted from T. Levett-Jones, K. Hoffman, Y. Dempsey, S. Jeong, D. Noble, C. Norton, J. Roche & N. Hickey (2010). The 'five rights' of clinical reasoning: an educational model to enhance nursing students' ability to identify and manage clinically 'at risk' patients. *Nurse Education Today, 30*(6), 515–520.